THE
100-UP EXERCISE

WITH ILLUSTRATIONS AND DIAGRAMS

DORMOUSE

Originally published in 1908

© This 2014 edition published in the United Kingdom by
Dormouse Press, an imprint of Guidemark Publishing Limited

ISBN 9780957670402

British Library Cataloguing in Publication Data. A catalogue record for this book
is available from the British Library.

www.dormousepress.co.uk

INTRODUCTION

THE WONDERFUL CAREER OF W G GEORGE

W G George, one of the most remarkable figures to appear on the running track, was born on September 9th, 1858, at Calne, in Wiltshire.

On leaving school in 1876, he was apprenticed to a pharmaceutical chemist at Worcester, his duties, as he narrates in the first chapter of this little book, compelling him to remain within doors the whole day, with but one hour's leave for recreation, desire to make the most of which led to the invention and development of the "100-Up" Exercise.

HIS FIRST APPEARANCE ON THE TRACK

From the very first George had always taken deep interest in athletics, and the announcement of a mile walking handicap to be held at Birmingham resulted in the future famous runner entering his name as a competitor in this, his one and only walking race. Started from the 45-yards mark, he made a dead heat. The "decider" looked like finishing in the same way, but as excitement among the onlookers increased, it infected the two contestants, until both broke into a run, sprinting the last 50 yards as hard as they could go; for which offence, however, they could not be disqualified as they were only competing for prizes already won.

HIS FIRST RUNNING MATCH

This was remarkable for two things: it was the last contest in which George was given a start—from the 45-yards mark; and after he had finished first in 4 minutes 29 seconds, he was objected to on the score of making too good a time for a novice; and it was suggested that he was a professional, running under an assumed name.

The race was the mile at the Notts Forest Football Sports held at Nottingham in 1877. After proper enquiries had been made, he was awarded the prize; but never again did he start in a race from anywhere but the scratch line, a record probably unique in racing annals.

SUBSEQUENT AMATEUR CAREER

After winning a mile handicap at Chesterfield on rough grass, from scratch in 4 minutes 31 seconds, George ran, in 1878, his first cross-country race, the Spartan Harriers' Novices' Steeplechase, over 5½ miles of country at Edmonton. He won comfortably, and this success was followed by a score or so of others at various distances from 440 yards up to 4 miles in different parts of the country. In the spring of the following year, 1879, he won the

One and the Four-mile Amateur Athletic Championships at Stamford Bridge, the former in 4 minutes 26⅕ seconds, the latter in 20 minutes 51⅘ seconds; and he took the same events in 1880 in 4 minutes 28⅖ seconds, and 20 minutes 45⅘ seconds.

In the same year, the Midland Counties Cross-country Championships of 10½ miles fell to him, and many prizes throughout the country.

HIS VICTORY OVER L E MYERS

Owing to an accident in the early part of 1881, George was unable to train. Notwithstanding this, he put in an appearance at the Midland and National Cross-country Championships and defended his ½- and 1-mile titles at the AAA Championships, but was beaten into second place in all four events.

It was now that the late L E Myers, the American crack, paid his first visit to this country, challenging George to the ½ mile, 1,000 yards, and 1,200 yards. George refused, offering to run the ½, ¾ and 1-mile, but Myers would not agree, and returned to America after carrying off all before him, including the 440-yards championship.

But no sooner did he arrive on the other side than he cabled that he would run the distances named by George, if the latter would cross to New York.

On receipt of the cable, George proceeded to the States, and met the redoubtable American. The ½-mile was won by Myers by 2 feet in 1 minute 56⅖ seconds. The ¾ and 1-mile were run at the Polo Grounds, New York, on Thanksgiving Day. George won the mile fairly comfortably in 4 minutes 21 seconds.

A GREAT AND MEMORABLE RACE

In the presence of between 50,000 and 60,000 spectators, George won the ¾-mile. But Myers remained favourite for the last and supreme test of the series. George took the lead at once, and held his place to the 1,000 yards post, when Myers tried to force himself to the fore; but George gave him no chance, and so they passed together into the home straight, both men dragging themselves along only by the utmost effort. Thus they struggled on until about 20 yards from the tape, when Myers fell insensible. George staggered through the tape, the winner of what had proved one of the most exciting races on record. He managed to walk to his dressing-room, but pitched headlong through the doorway, where he lay on the floor as insensible as Myers was on the track, and was only brought back to consciousness about two hours later. Yet neither man felt any the worse on the following day for his experience.

Returning home at Christmas, George met with a most enthusiastic reception, being feted and feasted at Worcester, Birmingham, and London, and honoured with presentations and addresses from all sides, for it had been the general opinion that Myers was unbeatable.

A "GEORGE" YEAR

Or rather a "By-George!" year was 1882, for our hero annexed the Midland and National Cross-country Championships, both from big fields, and by a margin of over a quarter of a mile, followed by the capture of a whole string of prizes, including several challenge cups, double and treble wins in the London district, Woodbridge, Birmingham, Worcester, Stourbridge, Kidderminster, Lewes, Tewkesbury, Stoke-on-Trent, Widnes and many other places. At the Championship Meeting held that year at Stoke-on-Trent, he accomplished the hat-trick by winning the ½-mile, the 1-mile, and the 4-mile championships on the Saturday; while on the following Monday he gained the 10 miles. He also ran in the 2-mile steeplechase on the Saturday, but had to stop at 1½ miles, when a certain winner and leading by 60 yards, through losing a shoe. This record of winning four championships at one meeting has never been equalled except by George himself, when he repeated the performance in 1884 at Birmingham, and put up a new record of 4 minutes 18⅓ seconds for the mile in one of them.

AS CYCLE CHAMPION

Among other races won by George during this eventful year may be mentioned a 2-mile bicycle scratch race between six representatives of Worcester and Hereford. George rode an old-time high machine, and the race was wheeled on a track made by the members of the Worcester Cycle Club with their own hands, George himself helping in laying the track of five laps to the mile without banking.

Two days later George ran at Widnes, and took the ½ and 1-mile scratch races; also the 2-mile handicap from scratch, making good times in all three races.

Several sprints and the 440 yards handicap fell to his lot during the year, and he was capable of running the 100 yards in about a yard under 11 seconds, the quarter in 51 seconds, the mile in 4 minutes 20 seconds, and 10 miles in considerably under 52 minutes, and these and other such-like performances he could put up almost any day in the week. One one occasion, for instance, he won a sprint handicap, a 50-guinea 600 yards challenge cup level race, and a 10-mile handicap from scratch on the same day at Birmingham; while at Lewes he competed in every event on the card, winning prizes in the sprint, hurdles, quarter and mile, and taking first place in the steeplechase and high jump. On another occasion, at Marlow, he won the 440-yards, ran second in the mile and took the steeplechase, all from scratch in very fast times.

But perhaps the most wonderful record of this very remarkable athlete was that which he accomplished one afternoon at the Aston Lower Grounds, Birmingham, in 1884, when in the annual match between Moseley and Blackheath Harriers, he won the ½-mile, the mile, and the 4-miles, and the 2-miles steeplechase, having as competitors in all four events picked men from all the best athletes of the day, meeting and beating fresh opponents in each race. The steeplechase came last in order. Wills of Oxford University had kept himself specially for this event, and was regarded as a certainty. George waited on him in the race, and though almost fagged out, kept within about 20 yards of him until the straight was reached. The water-jump was about 30 yards from the finish; and all the competitors had been jumping religiously into the water throughout the race. Wills cleared the hurdle, and for the last time took a ducking; but George made a supreme effort: he sprinted and leapt, clearing the hurdle and water, jumping well over 18 feet in all, and landed on the other side just as Wills was getting out of the water. Impetus carried George past the post, the winner of what was probably the grandest race and best performance of his extraordinary career.

During this same year, George put up new records for almost every distance from 1,000 yards up to 12 miles at Stamford Bridge, the London Athletic Club having arranged a series of handicaps run in the evenings to suit his convenience, afterwards presenting the incomparable runner with a magnificent 22-carat gold shield with all the records established by him engraved thereon.

1883

This was a particularly unfortunate year, the great athlete losing all six championships which he held. The reason for this was, undoubtedly, that in his eagerness to surpass his previous efforts, he over-trained and became stale. In the Midland Cross-country Championships he finished fifth; and in the National which followed he was a few yards behind G A Dunning. By the time the AAA championships were due he had recovered some of his old form; but did not enter for them, simply because, being the holder of the ½, 1, 4 and 10-miles, he claimed the right of free entry, which right the authorities saw fit to dispute. The matter led to special investigation, when the right of championship holders to free entry was acknowledged and established by the formation of a new rule.

George, meanwhile, had done no training, but in the spirit of pure sportsmanship came forward to defend his titles, although he would have been quite justified in declining to do so. Of course, the untrained champion was bound to meet defeat— in the ½-mile by W Birkett in 1 minute 58 seconds; in the mile by W Snook in 4 minutes 25⅖ seconds; and in the 4-miles by the same man in 20 minutes 37 seconds.

But George had the satisfaction later of meeting and beating his great opponent W Snook; firstly, at the South London Harriers' Sports in a ¾-mile level race, and then in a series of races fixed up between them, winning easily from him in the 1 and 2-miles.

Of George's wonderful performances in 1884, we have already spoken, and we will now pass to the reasons why he

TURNED PROFESSIONAL

The phenomenal success attending George's amateur days brought about a heated paper controversy as to the respective merits of the performances put up by W Cummings, of Paisley, and the subject of our sketch. Cummings was the professional distance champion of the day, and held the World's Mile Record of 4 minutes 16⅕ seconds, or more than 2 seconds better than the Amateur Record put up by George, and while the latter held the World's 10-miles Record of 51 minutes 20 seconds, and all the then amateur records between ¾ of a mile and 12 miles, Cummings' time for the 10 miles was slightly slower, although he held most of the professional records up to 12 miles.

Everyone interested in athletics appeared to want to see a match between these two men, and George wrote to the AAA for permission to run a series of three races at 1, 4 and 10 miles with Cummings, suggesting that they, the AAA, should collect and take charge of all monies falling to his lot from the gate receipts, etc, over the races until the conclusion of the series, when the whole sum of money so obtained should be given in his name to a charity to be named by him.

But the AAA, after holding several meetings, came to the conclusion that it was their duty not to grant the request.

Now as George had won everything possible in the amateur world, and was itching for a match with Cummings, he decided to throw over his amateur status. He, therefore, issued a challenge through the *Sporting Life* to run a series of races at 1, 4 and 10 miles, for £100 a side for each contest. Cummings promptly accepted, deposits were posted with the *Sporting Life,* articles signed, and forthwith, for the first time in his life, George went into strict training, choosing Surbiton for his headquarters.

The first race, the mile, was run in September, 1885, at Lillie Bridge, in the presence of over 20,000 spectators. George won the toss, chose the inside, and set out to make the running at his best pace. The track was loose and heavy, so that the runners dug holes in it as they ran. The first quarter took 58⅗ seconds, the half 2 minutes 1 second. George stuck to it, but was disconcerted to feel his foot touched by Cummings every time his leg was thrown up behind.

At the 1,000 yards Cummings went sailing along on the outside, and George's heart sank as he observed that his opponent was, to all appearance, running superbly and without effort, with hand low down, and as cool as the proverbial cucumber. But George would not be done; he sprinted, drawing away from Cummings, and at the ¾-mile was leading by yards—time 3 minutes 7½ seconds. Although well-nigh exhausted, he kept going, leaving the other further and further behind, until the latter gave up the chase.

CUMMINGS' LITTLE DODGE

It appeared that when Cummings drew level it was his expiring effort; and as this was George's first encounter with this redoubtable runner, he was unacquainted with the latter's easy-running action even when at the end of his tether; and George learnt also that the touches on his heels which had so perturbed him came from the tips of Cummings' fingers, it being a favourite trick of his thus to worry the man just in front of him.

When Cummings stopped, the shouts of the crowd drew George's attention to the state of affairs, and he slackened to a walk. Then Cummings started again, but George pushed home, which he reached in 4 minutes 20⅓ seconds. George himself is of the opinion that had Cummings kept going that day, he (George) would have made better time then than later when he put up his hitherto unbeaten world's mile record of 4 minutes 12¾ seconds.

A DISAPPOINTING CONTEST

The 4-miles race took place a fortnight later at the Powderhall Grounds, Edinburgh. It was raining in torrents, and the wind was like a hurricane; but as there were some 12,000 people present, postponement was out of the question.

George won the toss, and, taking into account the weather conditions, decided to make a waiting race of it. But Cummings had formulated the same plan, and would not go to the front, though George slackened his pace almost to a crawl for the first 1½ to 2 miles; the crowd becoming restive and then irritated, jeering the runners, until George, disregarding risks, let himself go and tried to get away. But Cummings, who had been sheltering himself under the lee of his bigger opponent, hung on until about three quarters of a mile from home, when he shot forward on the outside, and sprinting for all he was worth, he ran clean away, winning easily to his own astonishment and George's disgust at finding himself so completely out-manoeuvered.

THE TEN MILES

On returning to London to complete his training, everything seemed to go wrong with him. He was ill, fainting repeatedly for the first time in his life; no less than seven times, two days prior to the match. But, notwithstanding his state of ill-health, he appeared on the track, and took the lead at the start, but ran very slowly, taking 5 minutes 21 seconds for the first mile. Cummings dashed to the front at 1¼ miles and was never again headed, winning the race in 51 minutes 6⅗ seconds—a world's record at the time—beating George by about 350 yards. It is probable that George ran the best and gamest race of his life on that day, although he was beaten, for he was totally unfit to run. A remarkable feature of the race was that Cummings was very exhausted at the finish, and was very sick during the last lap, while George seemed to improve, and was running much fresher and faster at the finish than either he or his opponent had run at any previous period of the race.

And so ended George's first series of races as a professional. He was greatly dissatisfied with the result; not from a money point of view, but because he had been so badly beaten.

George now crossed to America, but it was some months before he had completely recovered his health and strength. He has never been able to discover the cause of his illness, but has a strong suspicion that he had been poisoned in some way or other.

While in the States he ran the late L E Myers three exhibition races in Madison Square Gardens. The track of eight laps to the mile was unsuited to George's long stride; but Myers would run on no other, so George gave way and was defeated in all three races.

RETURN MATCH WITH CUMMINGS

The spring of 1886 saw George back in England, when a second match was proposed and ratified between Cummings and himself for races of 1, 4 and 10 miles as before.

The first race took place at Lillie Bridge, West Brompton, on Monday evening, August 23rd, 1886. In the presence of some 20,000 spectators, George, having won the toss, dashed to the fore, followed by Cummings a few feet behind. The first quarter was covered in 58¼ seconds. The half-mile saw no alteration in the respective positions; time 2 minutes 2 seconds. Just before the ¾-mile post was reached, Cummings sprinted, and raced level with George, the two passing the ¾-mile post in 3 minutes 7¾ seconds. Now Cummings drew ahead until there was a gap between the runners of 6 to 8 yards.

The crowd was greatly excited, and shouts of "Cummings wins!" "10 to 1 on Cummings!" resounded on all sides. But George knew directly Cummings sprinted that it was a killing effort to make so far from home. On coming into the back straight, he let himself go a bit, gradually lengthening his stride and creeping up to Cummings until he had reduced the latter's lead to a yard.

Meanwhile the spectators had become almost frantic with excitement, and the waving and shouting were almost deafening. Rounding the first corner of the top straight, George drew level, and then slowly—very slowly—got ahead of him. Turning into the home straight, both men running the race of their lives, George gradually increased his lead until about 2 yards ahead, when, some 60 yards from home, Cummings collapsed and fell in a heap on the grass by the side of the track, a fact of which George was made aware only after passing the tape.

Time 4 minutes 12¾ seconds—The record for the mile, which has stood unbeaten and even unequalled to the present day.

As a spectator has written: "Everyone remained in their places, and a peculiar silence came over the crowd as it waited for the time to be displayed on the board; then what a roar went up—such a roar as thrills me even now as I write this. It was stupendous, and the scene that immediately afterwards ensued was something never to be forgotten, as the thousands broke loose from every quarter, and rushed madly across the grounds towards the victor. These frenzied spectators literally overwhelmed him, swarming round, shouting, yelling, dancing and jumping about like madmen. Those who got near him slapped and banged him on the back, yelling as they did so: 'Grand!' 'Splendid!' 'Glorious!' Thus they continued until all the little remaining breath in George's body was well-nigh beaten out of it."

On September 11th, 1886, the 4-mile race took place at Preston. There was a splendid attendance, and everyone anticipated a good race. Cummings won the toss, but gave George the inside position. The track was good, and the day favourable for fast time; but for some unaccountable reason, George "could not run a yard." He started slowly, finishing the first mile in 5 minutes 6⅕ seconds; 2 miles in 10 minutes 12⅖ seconds; and 3 miles in 15 minutes 28⅘ seconds. Here Cummings took up the running, and George could not go his pace, and had to stop, or rather did stop, and then went on again; but it was useless.

George has never yet satisfied himself why it was that he could not run in either of his two 4-mile races with Cummings; it is possible that he had trained most strictly for the mile on each occasion, and the 4-mile races came too soon after the decision of the mile contests to suit him. He wanted a longer time in which to adapt himself to the different sort of running required for the two different distances.

The 10-miles and final of the second series of races with Cummings took place at Aston Lower Grounds, Birmingham, on October 2nd, three weeks after his defeat at Preston in the 4-miles.

George took the lead at the start and was never headed, the times being (until the race was stopped and George was declared the winner):

1 MILE	4 minutes	45 seconds
2 MILES	9 minutes	40⅕ seconds
3 MILES	14 minutes	40⅕ seconds
4 MILES	19 minutes	51 seconds
5 MILES	25 minutes	4⅘ seconds
6 MILES	30 minutes	26⅘ seconds

The race was practically over at 3½ miles, for Cummings had to stop and readjust his elastic stocking at about this point, so that George lapped him, and again almost did so a second time at 6 miles, soon after which Cummings stopped and intimated that he had relinquished the contest. It was a bad ending to a good race, but one of those misfortunes quite unavoidable.

And so ended this race with Cummings, and George's active English athletic career. In all he had won nearly £5,000 as a professional, out of nine races—six with Cummings, and three with L E Myers. As an amateur, George annexed just over 1,000 prizes, totalling a value of £4,000, and during his career established records at every distance between 660 yards and 12 miles, besides running races from 100 yards up to 600 yards, and competing successfully in cycle races, hurdle and walking races, high jumps, and in sculling, tennis, fishing and shooting contests. Finally, in winning a total of twelve English amateur track championships during his career, he established a record which still holds good to this day.

THE "100-UP" EXERCISE
BY ITS INVENTOR, W G GEORGE

CHAPTER 1

ITS BIRTH AND HISTORY

With the invigorating action of walking and running as a basis, and designed for the purpose of providing a natural system of home-training exercise to be used as an adjunct to, or a substitute for, outdoor training and recreation, the "100-Up" Exercise should be known and practised by all.

Its birth was the outcome, on the one part, of a perforce curtailed opportunity for outdoor recreation, and, on the other part, of a craving for health-giving exercise such as the body and limbs had grown accustomed to from early boyhood.

It was when I became articled in 1874 to chemistry at Worcester, that, as an indoor apprentice, I first missed the freedom of the open air and the joy of outdoor exercise. My father loved the open country of the Wiltshire wilds and inculcated in his children a like passion; yet here was I, a youth of sixteen, cooped up, with the exception of one short hour's leave for recreation, from 7am to 9pm daily, after which—supper, one hour's study, and then to bed.

ITS INCEPTION AND DEVELOPMENT

Necessity is the mother of invention. My physique cried out for its accustomed exercise—the health-giving tonic which was denied it. The brain, alone remaining active, sought to alleviate the trouble, and, becoming convinced of the importance of the case, evolved the idea which, in a perfected form, is the "100-Up" Exercise of today—a system of home exercise and training now practised by thousands, all of whom swear by it.

I did not at once impart the knowledge of my invention to anyone, but proceeded to test its efficacy upon my own physique. I was more than surprised at the results. Continuing to experiment and improve on the bare idea, I was gratified to find myself as fit in bodily health—despite the long hours indoors—as I had formerly been, and, with the regaining of my normal health, there came improvement of the muscles and additional strength to the vital organs. This gave me every encouragement to persevere, and the crowning triumph came when, having been persuaded to enter into some competition or other, I sent my name in for a 1-mile race at Birmingham. Greatly to my surprise, I scored a success from the short handicap mark of 45 yards, without ever having had a stripped practice; and though I had never attended a sports meeting, or been on a track before.

TRAINING ON THE "100-UP"

This was not the only success I achieved by reason of the magic of my newly-discovered home exercise, persistently practised; for from that time onward, right through the first five or six years of my athletic career, during which time I carried off many prizes and won several championships, I was almost entirely dependent upon the "100-Up" Exercise for my training; and in the following years which saw the zenith of my success in the athletic field, it was always a valuable adjunct to, and important item of, the programme of my athletic preparation.

Convinced at the outset of its great merits, I attempted to introduce the system to brother athletics and colleagues; but the response, at first, was not at all encouraging.

"100-Up! No, George, old chap; I had enough of that exercise last night at the club. Stukeley beat me five games off the reel—had some awful flukes!" Or else it was: "Why, you know I don't go in for *sprinting!*"

To these worthy gentlemen and others, I explained that the "100-Up" had no relation to billiards, nor was it beneficial to sprinters alone, but that it was an antidote to wet-day gloom or other sad times, when the exhilaration of outdoor exercise was denied one. Further, that its regular practice, whether alone or in addition to other training preparation or exercise, made the weak strong and the strong even stronger. The sceptics were persuaded to try it, became convinced, and adopted it for all time. The knowledge of the "good thing" was spread, its benefits proclaimed, and now thousands of its devotees, in the ranks of whom will be found doctors of eminence, clergymen, professional men of all classes, sportsmen and athletes in all branches of sports and games, including many prominent physical culturists and a goodly number of members of the fair sex, daily use the "Exercise of the Century" as a means of keeping themselves physically fit.

You wish to become a "Centurion"? Then follow me through the succeeding pages.

CHAPTER 2

EFFECT ON THE MUSCLES AND PHYSICAL ORGANS

A study of the "100-Up" Exercise from a scientific point of view shows that it brings into play the entire muscular system, without creating an undue strain on any one particular set of muscles, organ or limb. The heart and the lungs are reasonably exercised, superfluous tissue is gradually reduced, and muscles are built up in form and strength by a course of *natural,* not forced, development.

The exercise is unique in its simplicity, reliable in its efficiency, and is a recreative pleasure. It is inexpensive (requiring no apparatus), is easily learned, and is lasting in its benefits. As an adjunct to the actual track, road, field or river work of the sportsman or athlete in active training, it is invaluable. As a means of keeping the non-competitive member of the community physically fit, it has no equal. It is therefore an exercise of all-round importance and value, not only to the sportsman, athlete, rowing man, cyclist, walker, jumper, footballer, cricketer, golfer, huntsman, jockey, etc etc, but to every young or old, weak or strong person; in fact, to all those desirous of improving their natural physique and bodily health, and attaining general self-comfort and fitness throughout life.

SO SIMPLE

Its simplicity lies in the fact that there are no elaborate charts of exercise to memorise, no apparatus requiring to be fixed and adjusted before commencing, no special costume needed to exercise in, and therefore the least modicum of excuse or possible deterrent to *regular* practice, either on the score of expense, lack of time or of opportunity for regularity in the performance of this exercise—not all one day and nothing the next—is essential, just as in any other form of training.

One does not need a spacious gymnasium or exercise ground for the "100-Up". It can be practised on any firm floor space of the area of not less than six feet square. Moreover, it is an exercise which is graded to suit all ages and constitutions—and for both sexes—as will be seen from later chapters.

CHAPTER 3

HOW AND WHERE TO PRACTISE

There are ideal, scarcely ideal and non-ideal conditions in connection with everything to which we put hand or foot in this world, be it exercise or recreation, work or play, business or sport. There is a proper time for exercise as well as an improper one—for instance, no sane person would attempt strenuous exercise immediately after a hearty meal, or when thoroughly tired or fagged out. The common sense of the student will dictate the most suitable time, or times, of the day in order aptly to meet the circumstances.

The "100-Up" Exercise should be performed in the open air—in the back garden, or failing this, in a room well-ventilated, the window or windows being open at the time in order to permit free passage of air.

The ideal dress is loose-fitting, so as not to hamper free movement. Boots or shoes are of course required outdoors, but, indoors, the practice may be done, if preferred, in the stockinged feet.

The time, or times, of day devoted to the exercise must depend, as before-mentioned, very largely upon the habits or necessities of the subject. I find many of my friends utilise it as an ante-breakfast stimulator, the sort of thing that, in conjunction with the morning tub, banishes sleep from the eyelids, loosens the limbs and sets the heart, lungs and brain working with healthy action, puts the stomach into good condition, and tunes up the system generally, so as to be ready and alert for the business of the day.

WHEN TO PRACTISE

Many others prefer, first of all, that the stomach shall have a "lining" before anything is attempted, no matter how modest, in the shape of exercise, and I am of this persuasion myself, being convinced that the majority of people would be all the better for some little nourishment wherewith to break their fast before engaging in any form of physical training.

The beauty of the "100-Up" is that it may be practised any time during the day within reason, without changing a garment, and anyone who will follow the hints given and instructions laid down in this pamphlet, will be under no difficulty in adapting for themselves a programme and timetable best suited to their opportunities, needs and constitution. When I first started, I *made* my opportunities. My enthusiasm overcame the handicap from which I suffered. I would perhaps be sent up to the warehouse floor for a particular size of bottle or some other store, an errand involving time. Here was a chance of getting through a portion of the "100-Up"—sometimes it would be 10 or 20, at other times 30 or 40—and this would happen many times during the long day. Opportunities occur to the majority of us to transform moments of idleness into a lifetime of robust health.

THE BENEFIT OF ENTHUSIASM

Remember that enthusiasm is requisite to the complete success of any health exercise or participation in sport, just as faith in medical treatment is half the battle in combating disease. Make of your training a pleasure, and it will store up unlimited joy and health for you.

Never overdo it by distressing or fagging yourself out. One should always proceed gradually. Therefore do not exceed in speed or length of duration that which is laid down in the schedule of conditions hereafter indicated. Regularity is the keynote that brings forth the magnificent chord of success; non-regularity is inexcusable with such a simple, ready-to-hand, few-minute exercise as the "100-Up".

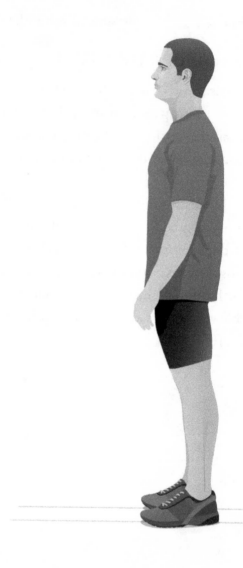

FIGURE 1

CHAPTER 4

PRELIMINARY PRACTICE FOR THE EXERCISE

Draw two parallel lines along the ground, 18 inches long and 8 inches apart.

Place one foot on the middle of each line. Stand flat-footed, the feet lying perfectly straight on the lines. The arms should be held naturally, loosely, and, except for a slight forward inclination, nearly straight (see Figure 1).

Now raise one knee to the height of the hip, as shown in Fig 2 (that is precisely in the same way as in walking, only the knee action is higher), and bring the foot back and down again to its original position, touching the line lightly with the ball of the foot. Repeat this exercise of raising and lowering the leg ten to thirty times. Then go through precisely the same performance with the other leg.

Practically, the foregoing amounts to balancing the body on one leg while exercising the other. Care must be taken that the knee comes up to the level of the hip every time. This may not be found easy at first, but practice will soon bring about the desired result. Every attention must be paid to keeping the body upright and the legs and feet quite straight while exercising. Practise slowly until the necessary balance is acquired and the exercise can be accomplished with ease. Otherwise the "100-Up" will be found unsatisfactory.

The preliminary practice as set out above is intended mainly for the purpose of preparing the leg muscles for the more severe strain required of them for the "100-Up" Exercise proper. It is the primary step in becoming a "Centurion".

A WARNING NOTE

I have said that the knee must be brought up to the level of the hip at each movement. Perhaps this is too much to ask from all who give the exercise a trial, for the "100-Up" is a general exercise in which all may participate, with advantage and benefit to themselves. What I mean is that the bringing up of the knee to the full height is the perfection stage, and the one which all users of the exercise should aim at; but it stands to reason that a very delicate or weakly youngster, an elderly person, or a fat individual of any age or either sex would find it impossible of accomplishment. To these I would say, raise the knee as high as convenience and comfort render possible of achievement, and set the mind and will on the ultimate accomplishment, little by little, of the perfection stage, i.e., the desired height. By dint of regular practice, the man or woman encumbered with too much fat will find the superfluous tissue gradually vanish; and the delicate or weakly person who at first can only lift the knee halfway will gradually be able to improve upon this, and subsequently reach the full height, by reason of the increased strength which the exercise will give to the muscles and physique generally.

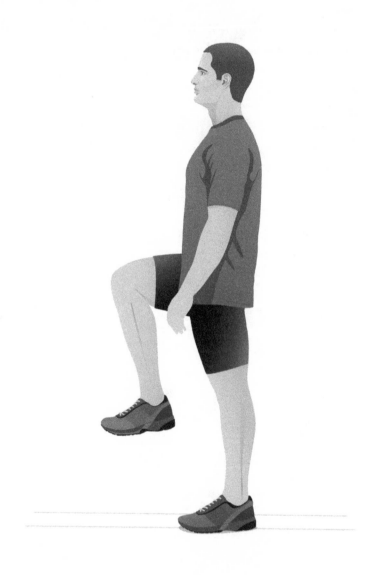

FIGURE 2

CHAPTER 5

THE "100-UP" EXERCISE PROPER

First of all, let me impress upon the student the necessity of maintaining perfect form in every practice, be it in the preliminary or in the exercise proper. Directly the correct form is lost the work should stop. Beginners should start the exercise slowly, and on no account strain or over-exert themselves. Hurried or injudicious training, or fast work while the system is unprepared for it, induces breakdown and failure. On the other hand, slow, well-considered, steady practice is never injurious, while breakdowns are practically unknown among those who start their training slowly, and who gradually increase distance, time or pace as the heart, lungs, and the muscular system throughout grow accustomed to the extra strain, and revel in it.

THE MINOR AND MAJOR GRADES

I have divided the "100-Up" Exercise into two grades—the Minor and the Major. The Minor is for all classes when learning, and is the limit for those who are physically incapable, through age or through infirmity, of particpating in the more strenuous or trying Major form of the exercise, which latter may be graduated, however, to suit the requirements of the individual. For instance, the student once having acquired the correct action, has two courses open to him or her. If he be an active athlete, he will naturally practise strenuously—and always correctly—and will adapt the length and pace of his bouts to suit and help the particular object, no matter what branch of sport it occurs in, that he has in view. But those who desire to perform the exercise for health and for the sake of longevity alone do not require to exercise more strenuously than circumstances warrant or permit; nor would it be wise for them to exact from the legs more than they can accomplish with benefit to those members and the whole body generally. The exact amount or extent of the exercise to prescribe for individual practice can only be apportioned by participants themselves; but every one should bear in mind that it is the exercise proper and perfect stage that he or she is attempting ultimately to perform.

THE MINOR EXERCISE

Prepare lines as for the preliminary practice. Stand on them as before. Hold the arms naturally and nearly straight, with a slight forward inclination (as in Figure 1).

Now raise one knee to the height of the hip, and bring the foot back and down again to its original position, touching the line lightly with the ball of the foot and repeat with the other leg (as in Figure 2). Continue raising and lowering the legs alternately. The main thing to remember is correct action. See

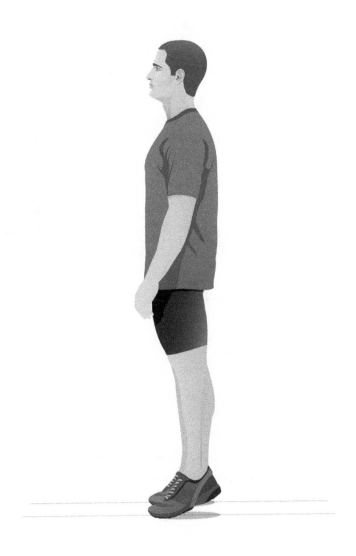

FIGURE 3

that the knees are brought up at each stride to the level of the hip if possible, or as near to this point as can be managed by the too-fat or bodily-infirm individual, and that the body maintains its correct perpendicular.

The exercise at first sight looks so easy of accomplishment that one might very well think it possible to go a thousand up. This is the result of not raising the knees to the prescribed height—the main point of the exercise—or of "galloping" through a short-timed movement in incorrect form. Get a friend to watch you at your practice and to correct any shortcomings in your leg action or poise of the body, and you will find the difference. No single part of the minor "100-Up" must be performed carelessly if the desired benefit is to result. Correct form once attained, the exercise may be increased in severity by gradually working from 10 to 20, 30 to 40, and so on up to the "100-Up" at each session, and by speeding-up the pace.

THE MAJOR EXERCISE

This exercise is more diffcult of accomplishment, yet comes easy to the student who by reason of having attained correct form in the preceding preparation will have, at the same time, acquired strength and the art of properly balancing the body when in action.

Stand on the lines marked on the ground as before, except that the body must be balanced on the ball of the foot, the heel clear of the ground, the head and the body being tilted very slightly forward, and the hands down by the side (see Figure 3).

Now spring from the toe, bringing the knee to the level of

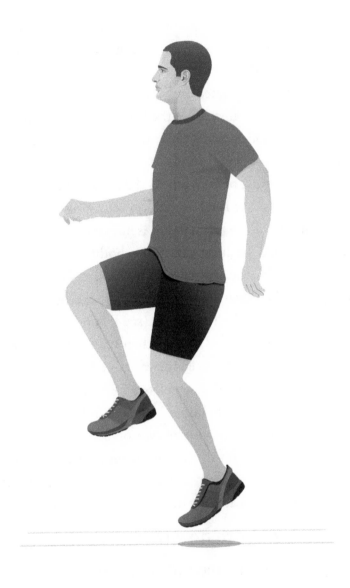

FIGURE 4

the hip or as near to that point as physique will permit, as in the minor exercise (see Figure 4), letting the foot fall back to its original position. Repeat with the other leg, and continue raising and lowering the legs alternately. This action is exactly that of running, except that instead of the legs moving forward as each stride or leg action is performed, the foot drops back into its original position on the ground.

The knees must be brought to the level of the hip (for full benefit) as each stride is taken, and on returning the foot to the ground, care should be taken that it is not carried further behind than the original position. Thus the body is practically kept upright except for the very slight tilt forward. When the knee is brought higher than level with the hip, the body is thrown out of its perpendicular backwards (see Figure 5) and when the foot is thrown out behind further than level with the back, the body is correspondingly forced forward (see Figure 6). These two pictures are intentionally exaggerated in order to illustrate the more plainly what I mean. Either fault is a hindrance to form and pace when in competition—the two objects which are striven for by those who train for running. A much greater amount of benefit will be derived from doing the practice correctly and in good form than by scamping it.

WHAT TO DO WITH THE ARMS

While performing the "100-Up" Major exercise, use the arms as they should be used in the correct way for running, i.e. hold them at full length and swing them forward half across the body and backwards a few inches behind the back as each stride is taken.

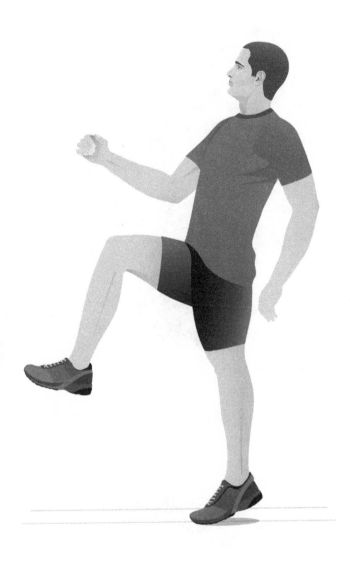

FIGURE 5

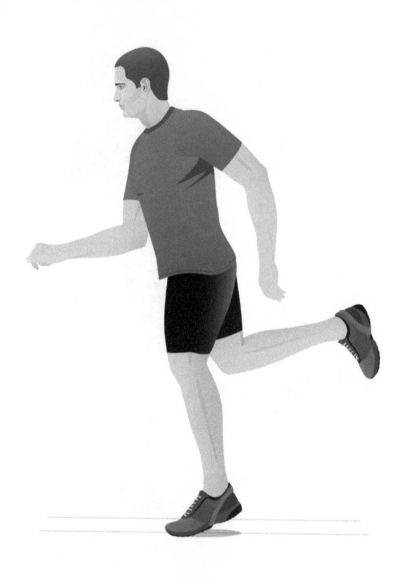

FIGURE 6

A good practice is to stand still on the lines and use the arms as in running, putting plenty of force into the work, so as to loosen the muscles of the shoulders and make the upper part of the frame active and pliable, in order that it may act in perfect union with the legs when the "100-Up" is performed—the object being to teach one the true and proper action of the arms in active competition.

ADVICE TO BEGINNERS

I do not advise anyone to attempt more than 20-Up of the exercise at the start, ten for each leg. Very few can manage so many in correct form at the outset, but regular practice brings greater stamina and an ease of action which renders the task less arduous, and once the 20-Up has been accurately accomplished, the number may be steadily increased. Let me say a word or two of warning, however, against too rapid a progress. This may result in a strain, or what is even more likely, a loss of correct form. The knees will not be parallel to the straight lines, or the body will be dragged forward, and this departure from the orthodox or correct form of the action will destroy the beauty of the movement and the greater part of the value of the exercise as a whole.

The student must not expect to get true action in a moment. The first few attempts may even be disappointing, but keep steadily on trying, and the correct form will come sure enough. Once having become proficient, he can keep on working gradually up to the "100", and by judicious variation of pace and number, the athlete can so frame his exercise as to suit the speed and stamina required for the competition, race or branch of sport he has in view, and about which I shall have something more to say in the following chapter.

CHAPTER 6

WHAT THE EXERCISE TEACHES

Proficiency having been attained in the performance of the "100-Up" Exercise, and its great possibilities realised, one is able to bring careful thought to bear on the subject of his or her own particular individual needs, whereby the greatest value may be extracted from the practice of the exercise as a means towards the acquisition of physical perfection. Most people will agree with me that discreet exercise or training is beneficial and conducive to a healthy existence and long life. A man or a woman who engages himself or herself exclusively to work or study, shunning all bodily exercise and pleasure, is but qualifying for martyrdom, in later years, to one or other of the ills to which flesh is heir.

FOR THOSE OF SEDENTARY HABITS

If as an ordinary citizen of somewhat sedentary occupation you wish to supplement the meagre amount of walking or other exercise for which you are able to find time, the "100-Up" is the very thing, and its regular practice, judiciously applied, will always keep you trim and in good order.

FOR SPORTSMEN

If, as a participator in active outdoor sport on intermittent occasions—such as at weekends, etc—you seek a means of keeping the muscles pliable, and the body in good condition for the fray, you cannot do better than daily indulge in the "Century" exercise, and you will be surprised at the improvement its practice will bring in your play or in the performance of any kind of sport or pastime to which you are addicted. It will always keep you in good form, ready to give of your best, be it in cricket, football, tennis, golf, rowing, hockey, boxing, hunting or other sport or pastime.

FOR ATHLETES

If, as an athlete in constant training, you wish in a natural way to improve the muscles, and more particularly to increase your stride to its greatest possible length without extra exertion, to attain perfect form and greater speed, to strengthen the vital organs and thus obtain greater stamina, the "100-Up" as part of your schedule of training-exercise will accomplish what you want, and give you your heart's desire. I have known an athlete to increase his stride by over 2 inches after a month's practice of the exercise, without once visting a track for training purposes during that time.

FOR GROWING LADS AND LASSES

If, as a growing youth or maid, you wish to attain good physique, pliability of limb and uprightness of carriage, the exercise, in its moderated form for the young and for those past middle age, gives excellent results without any violence of method.

FOR EVERYBODY

Not only is the "100-Up" a health exercise and muscle developer, but it also teaches the correct carriage of the body in walking and in running—ordinary or competitive—viz, the correct pose of the head and angle at which to carry the body; the right way in which to carry the legs and feet, and how to pick up and put down the latter; also the proper arm action.

CORRECT ACTION

To explain the correct way to walk or to run, I would say: The feet must be picked up from the ground in a perfectly clean manner; there must be no shuffling in the action. For this purpose, the legs and feet should be always held in a straight, forward line, not turned out or in, twisted or wobbled about in any way, either when they are carried through space, when in action or moving forward, or when the feet are actually on the ground itself.

This straight action helps to keep the body steady and upright, which is the acme of perfection, except when in actual running, when there should be the slightest tilt forward of the head and body, obviously necessary for the purpose of keeping the body in perfect balance while moving more or less rapidly forward.

In race walking or running, the feet should fall on the ground as each stride is taken in a straight line, thus:

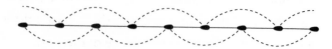

The markings denote faultless footmarks when race walking or running correctly, in contrast to

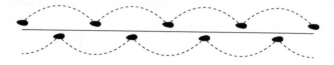

denoting bad form in running or walking. The "100-Up, properly practised, insures absolutely correct running action. The bringing up of the knee to the level of the hip in practice insures the longest individual stride-action possible of accomplishment in competition, although in running the knee is not brought up higher than just high enough to permit of the leg and foot to shoot out forward to their fullest extent before the ball of the foot comes in contact with the ground, from whence the next stride or spring is taken. The "Century" exercise teaches all this to perfection.

THE CORRECT POSE

The correct pose of the head and body in ordinary walking is upright, yet loose and supple. There should be nothing stiff or rigid in the carriage, yet there must not be any perceptible movement present except the forward one, and this should be performed in a uniform way, without jerk or jerkings of any kind throughout the whole length of the body during the movement.

The arms, both in walking and running, should be kept

almost at full length, and held down and loosely swung in perfect union with the legs as each stride is taken—the slight bending of the elbow and wrist necessary makes the forearm and hand act as a sort of lever or paddle, and assists the forward movement of the opposite leg in its endeavour to stride out its furthest as each step is taken. The "100-Up" will do all this for you if you have the will to make it do so.

CONCLUSION

Success is the result of the application of scientific methods of training to the development of natural talents or skill, which we all possess in some degree or other. In placing the "100-Up" exercise before the public, and thus spreading the knowledge of it still further, I am confident I am giving them an exercise which though simple and natural in practice and incapable of harm when practised discreetly, is second to none as a means of attaining, and retaining, physical fitness, and of developing the body, muscles, and health generally. It is an in and outdoor exercise, embracing all that is good in preparation for all kinds of outdoor sports and recreations, and can be made to adapt itself for any and every kind of emergency, but safe and true, training for competitive purposes, as well as for general health, perfect fitness and recreative amusement throughout life. By its constant practice and regular use *alone,* I have myself established many records on the running path, and won more amateur championships than any other individual has ever won in all times. Hence my supreme faith in what I honestly believe is the century's best—the "100-Up" Exercise.

CPSIA information can be obtained
at www.ICGtesting.com
Printed in the USA
BVHW03s1942100818
524132BV00001B/30/P